CONTENTS

Title: "Unlock Your Beauty Potential: The Ultimate Guide to Radiant Skin, Makeup Mastery, and Confident Style"

Author: Beauty Megbo

1

Introduction:

"Unlock Your Beauty Potential" is a comprehensive book that

encompasses a wide range of topics to help readers enhance their natural beauty, boost their confidence, and embrace their own unique style. With a holistic approach, Beauty Megbo offers expert advice, practical tips, and step-by-step instructions to help readers achieve radiant skin, master makeup techniques, and develop a confident and personalized style.

PART 1: RADIANT SKIN SECRETS

2. The Basics of Skincare

   - Identifying your skin type and specific needs

   - Developing a skincare routine for glowing skin

   - Addressing common skin concerns and conditions

3. Natural Beauty from Within

   - The importance of a balanced diet and hydration

   - Key nutrients for radiant skin

   - Incorporating skincare from your pantry

4. Skincare Rituals and Techniques

   - Step-by-step guide to daily cleansing, toning, and moisturizing

   - Exfoliation and skincare treatments

   - The benefits of face masks and facial massages

PART 2: MAKEUP MASTERY

5. Makeup Essentials for Every Skill Level

- Building a basic makeup kit

- Choosing the right foundation, concealer, and powders

- Exploring different makeup tools and brushes

6. Flawless Makeup Techniques

- Tips for achieving a natural, everyday look

- Mastering tricky techniques like contouring and highlighting

- Steps to create stunning eye makeup and brows

7. Makeup for Special Occasions and Beyond

- Creative and glamorous makeup looks for events

- Makeup for different seasons and trends

- Expert tips to make your makeup last all day

PART 3: CONFIDENT STYLE

8. Embracing Your Personal Style

   - Discovering your style personality

   - Tips for wardrobe organization and decluttering
   - Developing a signature style that reflects your personality

9. Dressing for Your Body Shape

   - Understanding different body types and proportions
   - Flattering clothing choices for your unique shape
   - Accessorizing to enhance your overall look

10. Building a Versatile Wardrobe

   - Smart shopping strategies for quality and budget
   - Essential wardrobe staples and how to mix-and-match
   - Creating different outfits for various occasions

Conclusion:

"Unlock Your Beauty Potential" is a comprehensive guide that equips readers with the knowledge and skills needed to enhance their natural beauty, master makeup techniques, and develop a confident personal style. Through the guidance and expertise of

Beauty Megbo, readers will be empowered to unlock their true beauty potential and usher in a new era of self-confidence and self-expression.

CHAPTER 1: INTRODUCTION TO UNLOCKING YOUR BEAUTY POTENTIAL

Introduction:

Beauty is not just about physical appearance; it encompasses a deeper, more profound connection between one's inner self and outer appearance. In this chapter, we will explore the fundamental concepts of unlocking your beauty potential by understanding the intricate link between inner and outer beauty. We will delve into the principles of self-acceptance and self-care, which are essential for nurturing and enhancing your unique beauty.

1.1 Understanding the Connection between Inner and Outer Beauty:

Beauty is not something that can be measured solely by external appearances. Instead, it is a reflection of a person's character, emotions, and overall well-being. Inner beauty radiates from within, influencing the way a person carries themselves, their outlook on life, and how they interact with others.

When inner beauty harmonizes with outer appearances, a person's true beauty potential is unlocked. It is crucial to understand that inner beauty is not something that can be solely nurtured through external means such as makeup or fashionable clothing. Rather, it requires a holistic approach that integrates physical, mental, and emotional well-being.

1.2 Embracing Self-Acceptance:

Self-acceptance is a vital component of unlocking your beauty potential. It involves embracing and appreciating your unique qualities, imperfections, and individuality. By acknowledging and accepting yourself, you can develop authentic confidence and radiate an alluring aura that transcends physical attributes.

Many individuals strive to meet societal beauty standards, often leading to dissatisfaction and a constant feeling of not being enough. However, self-acceptance allows individuals to embrace their true selves, fostering a positive self-image and healthier relationships with others. This chapter will guide you through various exercises and techniques to help you cultivate self-acceptance and love yourself unconditionally.

1.3 Practicing Self-Care:

Self-care is another fundamental aspect of unlocking your beauty potential. It involves nourishing your body, mind, and soul to promote overall well-being. Taking care of yourself not only enhances your physical appearance but also impacts your mental and emotional state.

In this chapter, we will explore various self-care practices, such as skincare routines, exercise, meditation, and fostering healthy relationships. These practices allow you to prioritize your needs and invest in your personal growth, leading to a more vibrant and beautiful you.

Conclusion:

Unlocking your beauty potential begins with understanding the connection between inner and outer beauty. Embracing self-acceptance and making self-care a priority are essential steps in this journey. By acknowledging your unique qualities, appreciating your individuality, and nurturing your mind, body, and soul, you can unlock the true essence of your beauty potential, radiating an irresistible glow that goes beyond physical appearances. In the following chapters, we will delve deeper into various aspects of unlocking your beauty potential and provide practical tips and guidance to help you along your transformative journey.

CHAPTER 2: PART 1 - RADIANT SKIN SECRETS

Introduction:

Achieving radiant skin goes beyond simply applying skincare products. It requires understanding your skin type, tailoring a skincare routine to address specific needs, and addressing common skin concerns and conditions. In this chapter, we will explore the basics of skincare, offering insights and practical advice to help you unlock the secrets to radiant skin.

2.1 Identifying Your Skin Type and Specific Needs:

Understanding your skin type is paramount in creating an effective skincare routine. Whether you have oily, dry, combination, or sensitive skin, each type requires a different approach to address its specific needs. This section will guide you through identifying your skin type and provide tips on how to care for it.

Additionally, we will delve into the various factors that affect your skin's health and appearance, such as genetics, environment, and lifestyle choices. By gaining insights into these influences, you will be able to develop a personalized skincare routine that caters to your unique requirements.

2.2 Developing a Skincare Routine for Glowing Skin:

A well-crafted skincare routine is the foundation for achieving and maintaining radiant skin. This section will outline the essential steps in a skincare routine, including cleansing, exfoliating, toning, moisturizing, and protecting your skin from harmful UV rays.

We will also explore the role of specialized skincare products, such as serums, masks, and eye creams, in addressing specific concerns like aging, hyperpigmentation, or acne. By incorporating these products into your routine, you can optimize the health and appearance of your skin, revealing a radiant complexion.

2.3 Addressing Common Skin Concerns and Conditions:

Even with a diligent skincare routine, various skin concerns and conditions may arise. This section will provide a comprehensive overview of common issues, including acne, dryness, sensitivity, and uneven skin tone.

You will discover helpful tips and remedies to address these concerns, including natural ingredients, lifestyle adjustments, and targeted treatments. By understanding how to approach and manage these challenges, you can enhance the overall health and beauty of your skin.

Conclusion:

Radiant skin is not elusive; it can be achieved by understanding your skin type, developing a skincare routine tailored to your needs, and addressing common skin concerns and conditions. By identifying your skin type and catering to its specific requirements, you lay the foundation for healthy and glowing skin.

In the next chapters, we will expand on these concepts, offering in-depth knowledge on specific skincare ingredients, advanced techniques, and expert advice from dermatologists to guide you on your journey to radiant skin. With dedication, consistency, and the knowledge gained from this chapter, you will uncover the secrets to achieving your desired skin goals.

13

CHAPTER 3: NATURAL BEAUTY FROM WITHIN

Introduction:

While skincare products play a vital role in achieving radiant skin, true beauty also comes from within. This chapter focuses on how your diet and hydration can significantly impact the health and appearance of your skin. We will explore the importance of a balanced diet, key nutrients for radiant skin, and how you can incorporate skincare from your pantry.

3.1 The Importance of a Balanced Diet and Hydration:

Your skin reflects your overall health and well-being, making a balanced diet crucial for radiant skin. This section will emphasize the significance of nourishing your body with a wide variety of nutrients, including vitamins, minerals, healthy fats, and antioxidants. We will delve into the benefits of consuming a colorful array of fruits and vegetables, lean proteins, whole grains, and avoiding excessive sugar and processed foods.

Additionally, adequate hydration is essential for maintaining skin health. We will discuss the impact of water intake on skin hydration, the signs of dehydration to watch out for, and tips for incorporating more fluids into your daily routine.

3.2 Key Nutrients for Radiant Skin:

Certain nutrients have a profound effect on the health and appearance of your skin. In this section, we will explore those key nutrients, such as omega-3 fatty acids, vitamin C, vitamin E, and zinc. You will learn how these nutrients contribute to collagen production, skin elasticity, and protection against free radicals.

To optimize your intake of these essential nutrients, we will provide a list of food sources that are abundant in each. By incorporating these foods into your diet, you can nourish your skin from the inside out.

3.3 Incorporating Skincare from Your Pantry:

Your kitchen holds a treasure trove of ingredients that can enhance your skincare routine. In this section, we will introduce various pantry staples that have proven benefits for the skin. These include natural ingredients like honey, avocado, oatmeal, turmeric, and green tea.

You will discover recipes and DIY skincare treatments using these ingredients, allowing you to create nourishing masks, scrubs, and infusions that will improve your skin's health without harsh chemicals or additives. We will also discuss the importance of patch testing and proper application techniques when using homemade skincare treatments.

Conclusion:

Achieving radiant skin doesn't solely rely on external products; it requires nurturing from within as well. By adopting a balanced diet, staying hydrated, and incorporating skincare from your pantry, you can provide your skin with the nourishment it needs to glow from the inside out.

In the following chapters, we will delve into advanced topics, such as mindful eating, Ayurvedic practices, and the role of gut health in skin appearance. By combining the knowledge gained from this chapter with a holistic approach, you will unlock the secrets to natural beauty and radiant skin.

CHAPTER 4: SKINCARE RITUALS AND TECHNIQUES

Introduction:

Building a consistent skincare routine is essential for maintaining healthy and glowing skin. This chapter will take you through the step-by-step process of daily cleansing, toning, and moisturizing. We will also explore the benefits of exfoliation, skincare treatments, face masks, and facial massages in achieving radiant and youthful skin.

4.1 Step-by-Step Guide to Daily Cleansing, Toning, and Moisturizing:

Proper cleansing, toning, and moisturizing are the foundations of any skincare routine. In this section, we will provide a detailed step-by-step guide to help you achieve clean and hydrated skin. You will learn about the different types of cleansers suitable for various skin types and techniques to effectively remove dirt, makeup, and impurities.

We will then move on to the importance of toning and selecting the right toner for your skin. You will discover the benefits of toning, such as restoring pH balance and tightening pores. Finally, we will explore the significance of moisturizing, including how to choose the right moisturizer and the proper application techniques for maximum hydration and protection.

4.2 Exfoliation and Skincare Treatments:

Exfoliation is a vital step in any skincare routine as it removes dead skin cells and promotes cell turnover, leading to a smoother and more radiant complexion. In this section, you will learn about different exfoliation methods, including physical and chemical exfoliants. We will discuss the frequency of exfoliation and how to avoid over-exfoliation, which can cause skin sensitivity.

Furthermore, we will delve into the world of skincare treatments, such as serums, essences, and ampoules. You will understand how these concentrated formulations can target specific skin concerns, such as fine lines, dark spots, and uneven texture. We will also discuss the proper order of applying these treatments within your skincare routine.

4.3 The Benefits of Face Masks and Facial Massages:

Face masks have become popular in recent years for their ability to provide deep hydration, nourishment, and intensive treatment to the skin. In this section, we will explore the different types of face masks, including sheet masks, clay masks, and gel masks. We will discuss their unique benefits and the recommended frequency of usage for each.

Additionally, facial massages offer numerous benefits for the skin, including improved blood circulation, lymphatic drainage, and relaxation. We will introduce various facial massage techniques and how they can stimulate collagen production, reduce puffiness, and enhance product absorption.

Conclusion:

Developing a skincare routine that encompasses daily cleansing, toning, and moisturizing is essential for maintaining healthy and radiant skin. In addition, incorporating exfoliation, skincare treatments, face masks, and facial massages can take your skincare routine to the next level, allowing for a rejuvenated and youthful complexion.

In the following chapters, we will dive deeper into targeted skincare concerns, such as acne, hyperpigmentation, and aging. By incorporating the knowledge gained from this chapter, you will be able to customize your skincare rituals and te

chniques to address your specific skin needs, resulting in healthier and more beautiful skin.

PART 2: MAKEUP MASTERY

Introduction:

Makeup has the power to enhance one's natural beauty and boost confidence. In this section, we will cover makeup essentials for every skill level. Whether you are a beginner or a seasoned makeup enthusiast, we will guide you through building a basic makeup kit, choosing the right foundation, concealer, and powders, as well as exploring different makeup tools and brushes.

5.1 Building a Basic Makeup Kit:

A well-rounded makeup kit is essential for creating various looks and catering to different occasions. In this section, we will provide a comprehensive list of makeup essentials that every beginner should have. From foundation to lipstick, eyeshadow palettes to mascara, we will cover the essentials that will allow you to experiment and discover your personal style.

We will discuss the importance of understanding your skin tone and undertones when selecting foundation and concealer shades. Furthermore, we will explore the various types of makeup brushes and their uses, ensuring that you have the right tools to achieve a flawless application.

5.2 Choosing the Right Foundation, Concealer, and Powders:

Foundation serves as the base for your makeup, creating an even canvas and blurring imperfections. In this section, we will guide you through choosing the right foundation formula, coverage, and finish for your skin type and desired look. We will also discuss the importance of shade matching and provide tips on how to find your perfect match.

Concealer is a versatile product that helps to cover dark circles, blemishes, and discoloration. We will explain the different types of concealers, such as liquid, cream, and stick, and how to properly apply them for a seamless finish.

Additionally, we will explore the role of powders in setting your makeup, controlling shine, and providing a smooth, matte finish. We will discuss the different types of powders, including translucent, pressed, and loose, and how to incorporate them into your routine for long-lasting wear.

5.3 Exploring Different Makeup Tools and Brushes:

Having the right makeup tools and brushes can make a significant difference in the application and final outcome of your makeup look. In this section, we will introduce you to various makeup tools, such as beauty blenders, makeup sponges, and brushes.

We will discuss the different shapes and materials of brushes and their specific functions, from foundation brushes to eyeshadow brushes. You will learn how to choose the right brushes for each step of your makeup routine and understand the importance of proper brush care for longevity and hygiene.

Conclusion:

Makeup mastery is within reach for anyone, regardless of their skill level. By building a basic makeup kit, choosing the right foundation, concealer, and powders, and exploring different makeup tools and brushes, you will be equipped with the necessary knowledge and products to create stunning makeup looks.

In the following chapters, we will further expand on specific makeup techniques, such as creating a flawless base, mastering eyeshadow application, and perfecting lip makeup. By incorporating the knowledge gained from this section, you will be able to elevate your makeup skills and express your creativity with confidence.

6. Flawless Makeup Techniques

Introduction:

In this section, we will delve into the art of flawless makeup techniques. Whether you want to achieve a natural everyday look or master more advanced techniques like contouring and highlighting, we've got you covered. Additionally, we will guide you through the steps to create stunning eye makeup and perfectly groomed brows.

6.1 Tips for Achieving a Natural, Everyday Look:

Sometimes, less is more, and a natural makeup look can be just as captivating as a more dramatic one. We will provide you with tips and tricks to achieve a flawless, natural look that enhances your features without looking overly done.

We will cover the importance of skincare as the foundation of any makeup look and discuss how to prep and prime your skin for a smooth, natural finish. Additionally, we will explore the techniques for creating a fresh-faced complexion, subtly defined eyes, and a natural-looking flush of color on the cheeks and lips.

6.2 Mastering Tricky Techniques like Contouring and Highlighting:

Contouring and highlighting are transformative techniques that can sculpt and add dimension to your face. In this section, we will demystify these techniques and guide you through the steps to achieve a perfectly chiseled look.

You will learn about the different types of contouring products and shades, as well as how to choose the right shades for your skin tone. We will provide detailed instructions on where and how to apply contour products to define your cheekbones, jawline, and nose, creating the illusion of structure.

Furthermore, we will discuss the art of highlighting, emphasizing the areas of your face you want to bring forward and create a luminous glow. You will learn about the types of highlighters available and how to apply them strategically for a radiant finish.

6.3 Steps to Create Stunning Eye Makeup and Brows:

The eyes are often considered the focal point of a makeup look, and properly enhancing them can make all the difference. In this section, we will guide you through the steps to create stunning eye makeup looks and perfectly groomed brows.

We will cover everything from selecting the right eyeshadow colors and finishes to suit your eye shape to blending techniques and creating depth and dimension. You will learn how to create both subtle everyday eye makeup looks and more daring, impactful looks for special occasions.

Furthermore, we will delve into the world of eyebrow grooming and shaping. You will discover different methods of defining and filling in your brows, such as using brow pencils, powders, or gels, depending on your preferences and desired outcome. We will also provide tips for achieving symmetrical brows and maintaining their shape.

Conclusion:

Flawless makeup techniques are the key to achieving a polished and professional look. By mastering tips for achieving a natural, everyday look, learning tricky techniques like contouring and highlighting, and following the steps to create stunning eye makeup and brows, you will be equipped with the knowledge and skills to elevate your makeup game.

Remember, practice makes perfect, and with time and dedication, you will become more confident in creating a flawless makeup look to suit your style and personality. In the following sections, we will further explore advanced makeup techniques, such as creating the perfect pout and experimenting with different makeup trends.

7. Makeup for Special Occasions and Beyond

Introduction:

In this section, we will discuss how to create creative and glamorous makeup looks for special occasions. Whether it's a wedding, prom, or a formal event, we will provide you with inspiration and step-by-step instructions to help you achieve stunning makeup looks that will turn heads.

7.1 Creative and Glamorous Makeup Looks for Events:

Special occasions call for extraordinary makeup looks that reflect your unique style and enhance your natural beauty. We will take you through various makeup styles suitable for different events, from elegant and classic to bold and avant-garde.

We will explore color schemes, techniques, and products that will help you create stunning evening looks. Whether you prefer a smoky eye, a glittery lid, or a statement lip, we will guide you on how to execute these looks flawlessly. Additionally, we will provide tips on choosing the right makeup for specific events, considering factors like lighting and dress code.

7.2 Makeup for Different Seasons and Trends:

As the seasons change, so do makeup trends. In this section, we will discuss how to adapt your makeup routine to the different seasons, incorporating the latest trends.

We will cover topics such as transitioning from a fresh and dewy spring look to a bronzed and glowy summer appearance. We will also explore the warm and earthy tones of fall, as well as the bold and vibrant shades of winter. You will learn how to incorporate seasonal colors into your makeup routine and create looks that complement the time of year.

Additionally, we will discuss the current makeup trends, such as glossy lids, monochromatic looks, or graphic eyeliner, and provide tips on how to incorporate them into your style.

7.3 Expert Tips to Make Your Makeup Last All Day:

There is nothing worse than spending time creating a flawless makeup look, only to have it fade or smudge as the day goes on. In this section, we will share expert tips and tricks to ensure your makeup stays put and lasts all day long.

We will discuss the importance of skincare as a base for long-lasting makeup and guide you through a skincare routine that will help your makeup adhere better. Additionally, we will provide recommendations for long-wearing foundation, setting powders, and setting sprays that will lock your makeup in place.

Furthermore, we will share techniques for preventing smudging and creasing, as well as touch-up strategies to keep your makeup looking fresh throughout the day or evening.

Conclusion:

Special occasions provide an opportunity to experiment with creative and glamorous makeup looks that go above and beyond your everyday routine. By exploring different makeup styles suitable for events, adapting your makeup to the seasons and trends, and implementing expert tips to make your makeup last, you will be ready to dazzle on any special occasion.

Remember to have fun and express your unique personality through your makeup choices. With the knowledge and skills gained from this section, you will be able to create stunning looks that leave a lasting impression. In the following sections, we will explore other facets of makeup, such as skincare, makeup for different skin types, and tips for enhancing your natural features.

PART 3: CONFIDENT STYLE

Introduction:

In this section, we will explore how to embrace your personal style and develop a confident sense of fashion. From discovering your style personality to organizing your wardrobe, we will provide you with tips and advice to help you feel comfortable and stylish in your own skin.

8. Embracing Your Personal Style:

One of the keys to confident style is understanding and embracing your personal style. In this section, we will guide you through the process of discovering your style personality. We will discuss different style archetypes and help you identify which one resonates with you the most.

We will explore various aspects of personal style, such as color preferences, clothing silhouettes, and patterns. By understanding what you love and what makes you feel confident and comfortable, you can start building a wardrobe that truly reflects who you are.

8.1 Tips for Wardrobe Organization and Decluttering:

A cluttered and disorganized wardrobe can make it challenging to create stylish outfits and navigate your daily fashion choices. In this part, we will provide you with practical tips and strategies for organizing and decluttering your wardrobe.

We will guide you through the process of sorting and categorizing your clothes, helping you identify what items to keep, donate, or discard. Additionally, we will provide tips for maximizing your closet space and arranging your clothes in a way that is efficient and visually appealing.

By decluttering and organizing your wardrobe, you will have a clear view of what you own, making it easier to create stylish outfits that reflect your personal style.

8.2 Developing a Signature Style:

De

veloping a signature style is a powerful way to express your individuality and confidence. In this section, we will discuss how you can develop a signature style that reflects your personality.

We will delve into the elements of a signature style, such as color palettes, key wardrobe pieces, and accessorizing. We will encourage you to experiment with different styles and find ways to incorporate elements you love into your everyday outfits.

We will also provide tips on how to curate a versatile wardrobe that can be easily mixed and matched to create a variety of looks. By developing a signature style, you will feel more self-assured in your fashion choices and radiate confidence to those around you.

Conclusion:

Confident style is all about embracing your personal preferences and developing a sense of fashion that reflects who you are. By discovering your style personality, organizing your wardrobe, and developing a signature style, you will be well on your way to feeling confident and stylish every day.

Remember, fashion is a form of self-expression, so don't be afraid to experiment and have fun with your style. Take the time to understand what makes you feel your best and create a wardrobe that truly represents your unique personality. In the following sections, we will explore additional facets of confident style, such as dressing for different body types and occasions, as well as tips for accessorizing and maintaining your clothes.

9. Dressing for Your Body Shape:

Introduction:

Understanding your body shape and dressing in a way that flatters your unique proportions is essential for confident style. In this section, we will guide you through the process of identifying your body type and provide tips on how to dress to enhance your best features.

9.1 Understanding Different Body Types and Proportions:

There are several common body types, including hourglass, pear, apple, rectangle, and inverted triangle. In this part, we will explain the characteristics of each body type, helping you identify which category you fall into.

We will explore the concept of proportions, emphasizing the importance of balancing your upper and lower body and creating a visually pleasing silhouette. By understanding your body type and proportions, you can make more informed choices when it comes to selecting clothing styles that emphasize your best features.

9.2 Flattering Clothing Choices for Your Unique Shape:

Once you have identified your body type, it is time to explore clothing choices that flatter your shape. In this section, we will provide you with tips on how to accentuate your assets and downplay any areas you may feel less confident about.

We will discuss different types of clothing styles, such as A-line dresses, structured blazers, and high-waisted jeans, that work well for specific body types. We will also highlight the importance of proper fit and tailoring, as well as choosing fabrics that drape and flatter your figure.

By understanding which clothing styles work best for your body type, you can create a stylish and flattering wardrobe that boosts your confidence and makes you feel amazing in your own skin.

9.3 Accessorizing to Enhance Your Overall Look:

Accessories play a crucial role in enhancing your overall look and adding a personal touch to your style. In this part, we will discuss various ways to accessorize to complement your outfit and highlight your unique personality.

We will explore different types of accessories, such as statement jewelry, belts, scarves, and handbags, and provide tips on how to choose the right accessories for your body shape and personal style. Additionally, we will discuss the art of layering accessories to create interesting and cohesive looks.

By mastering the art of accessorizing, you can elevate even the simplest outfit and make a fashion statement that is uniquely yours.

Conclusion:

Dressing for your body shape and choosing flattering clothing styles and accessories is a vital aspect of confident style. By understanding your body type, proportions, and selecting clothing and accessories that enhance your features, you can create a wardrobe that makes you look and feel fantastic.

Remember, fashion is about celebrating your individuality and feeling confident in your own skin. Embrace your body shape, experiment with different styles, and have fun expressing your personal style through clothing and accessories. In the following sections, we will dive deeper into tips for dressing for different occasions, such as formal events or casual outings, as well as provide suggestions for maintaining your clothes and expressing your style through grooming and beauty choices.

10. Building a Versatile Wardrobe:

Introduction:

Building a versatile wardrobe is essential for maximizing your style options and getting the most out of your clothing. In this section, we will guide you through smart shopping strategies, highlight essential wardrobe staples, and provide tips on creating different outfits for various occasions.

10.1 Smart Shopping Strategies for Quality and Budget:

When it comes to building a versatile wardrobe, it's important to be strategic with your shopping. In this part, we will provide you with smart shopping strategies to help you make the most of your budget while ensuring you invest in quality pieces that will last.

We will discuss the importance of understanding your personal style and lifestyle when making purchasing decisions. Additionally, we will provide tips on identifying high-quality fabrics, finishes, and construction techniques to ensure you are making wise investments.

Furthermore, we will touch on budget-friendly options such as shopping sales, thrifting, and exploring affordable brands without compromising on quality. By employing these strategies, you can build a versatile wardrobe within your budget.

10.2 Essential Wardrobe Staples and How to Mix-and-Match:

To create a versatile wardrobe, it's crucial to have a foundation of timeless and versatile pieces. In this section, we will discuss essential wardrobe staples that serve as building blocks for a variety of outfits.

We will guide you through the basics such as a well-fitting pair of jeans, a little black dress, tailored blazers, classic white shirts, versatile skirts, and comfortable yet stylish footwear. We will also discuss how these staples can be mixed-and-matched to create different looks for various occasions.

By investing in these key pieces and learning how to combine them creatively, you can create numerous outfits suited for work, casual outings, or formal events, without the need for excessive shopping.

10.3 Creating Different Outfits for Various Occasions:

Versatility in your wardrobe extends beyond mixing and matching basic pieces. In this part, we will provide tips on creating different outfits for specific occasions, including work, social events, and travel.

We will discuss how to transition your wardrobe from day to night with simple tweaks and accessories. We will also touch on the importance of investing in a few statement pieces that can elevate any outfit, such as a stylish blazer or a versatile dress.

By understanding how to adapt your wardrobe to different occasions, you can feel confident and appropriately dressed for any situation without needing a vast collection of clothes.

Conclusion:

Building a versatile wardrobe requires thoughtful shopping strategies, essential wardrobe staples, and creativity in outfit creation. By following smart shopping tactics, investing in quality pieces, and understanding how to mix-and-match your wardrobe, you can create numerous outfits suited for various occasions without breaking the bank.

Remember, versatility doesn't mean sacrificing your personal style. Embrace your unique taste and express yourself through the combinations and accessories you choose. With a versatile wardrobe, you will always have the perfect outfit at hand, empowering you to step out with confidence and style.